D1113515

# You Are
# STRONGER
## Than You Know

# You Are
# STRONGER
# Than You Know

...words of hope
and encouragement
for someone living with
chronic illness

Edited by Becky McKay

**Blue Mountain Press**™
Boulder, Colorado

We wish to thank Susan Polis Schutz for permission to reprint the following poems that appear in this publication: "So many choices…" and "Learning to accept and live with limitations…." Copyright © 2016 by Stephen Schutz and Susan Polis Schutz. All rights reserved.

Library of Congress Control Number: 2015954780
ISBN: 978-1-59842-980-0

▉ and Blue Mountain Press are registered in U.S. Patent and Trademark Office.
Certain trademarks are used under license.

Acknowledgments appear on page 92.

Printed in China.
First Printing: 2016

✺ This book is printed on recycled paper.

This book is printed on paper that has been specially produced to be acid free (neutral pH) and contains no groundwood or unbleached pulp. It conforms with the requirements of the American National Standards Institute, Inc., so as to ensure that this book will last and be enjoyed by future generations.

# Blue Mountain Arts, Inc.
P.O. Box 4549, Boulder, Colorado 80306

# Contents

(Authors listed in order of first appearance)

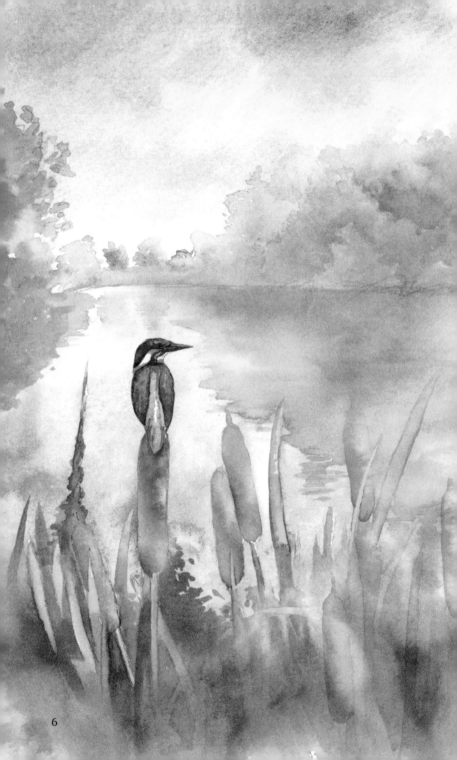

# You Are Stronger
# Than You Know

When we go through life's struggles, we sometimes feel weak. It is as if we have forgotten the many things we have been through and how we have changed our lives before.

At this very moment, no matter what you are going through… you are stronger than you know.

Sometimes we don't know our power until the time comes to use it. It lies dormant within us and emerges just when we think we can't go on. And when it does, we find that we had much more power and strength than we ever thought possible.

So when you feel like giving up and throwing in the towel, know in your heart that your strength is on its way to the surface. One day you will look back at this moment and see just how strong you really were.

You are stronger than you feel and much stronger than you know.

— Lamisha Serf-Walls

# A Little Pep Talk

Repeat after me:
I am strong.
I am special.
I can do anything.

Sometimes life throws
hurdles in our path,
but we just have to
keep on going
full speed ahead,
looking inside ourselves
for the courage
to leap over them
and never look back.

You are a strong
and remarkable person,
and you can do anything.
May you always
believe in yourself.

— Natalie Evans

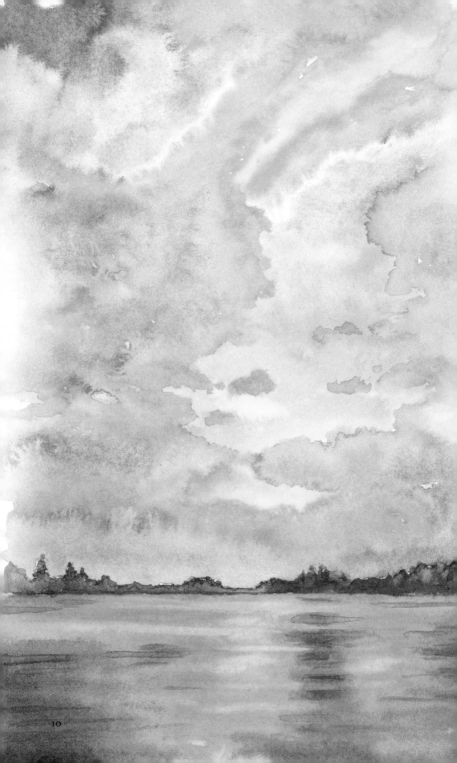

# Don't Let Your Circumstances Dull Your Spirit

As you dodge the curve balls that are coming at you now, don't let anything take away your hope, get you down, or make you give up. While you face these problems that touch the land mines in your soul, don't let them steal your power.

Stay strong, encouraged, and hopeful. Refresh your spirit with the lessons you've learned. You know your heart. You know who you are. There will be answers. Just be patient. Be satisfied with doing the best you can. When you're down, don't stay there. And never, never forget what a special person you are.

— Donna Fargo

# Know That You Are Never Alone

You may think you are
    alone at the moment,
and you may feel as if
    you are just soldiering on.
But you couldn't be more wrong,
because you have a whole army
    of people behind you.

So the next time you feel alone
    with your problems
or feel downhearted in any way,
remember that army of supporters
    behind you —
people who care about you
    and are wishing you well.

— Maria Mullins

# Draw Strength
# from Yourself and
# Your Surroundings

When the challenges seem so much greater than your strength, you may wonder how you will get through this day or even this hour. At times like these you need to look back to past trials and tribulations that you have gone through and survived. Remember them? The same strength that enabled you to get through those earlier storms is still within you. Reach down deep and draw from this wellspring; allow it to replenish your soul.

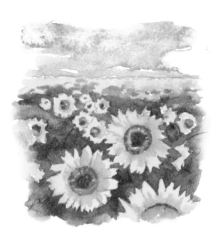

Borrow strength from others — those "warriors" who have already fought and won the battles you are struggling with today. Rejoice in their victories; they are with you in spirit. Draw strength from those who are with you in the battle today, for none of us truly walk alone.

Draw strength from the good things in your life — from the simplest to the greatest. Whether it's a pretty little flower, a kind word from a friend, a walk in your favorite place, or a beautiful sunset — draw strength from anything good that touches your heart or your day.

Draw strength from those who love you — those who make your life richer by being a part of your days, those who will be there for you not only on sunny days but also on the cloudy ones, and those who will hold you in the storms of life.

Have faith in yourself. Draw strength from your faith. And know in your heart that, just as before, this time will pass — because you have strength for today.

— Nancye Sims

# What It Means
# to Live with Illness

*I*llness, especially when it's invisible, makes us question everything that is familiar, socially acceptable, and comfortable.

*Illness makes us re-examine* our entire life, its priorities, meaning, and legacy.

*Illness strips us* of who we are, or at least who we perceive ourselves to be.

*Illness leaves us exposed and naked*, because everything familiar is now a potential enemy.

*Illness forces us* to delve into deeper layers, extracting the ideals we were raised with — ideals that hinder our emotional, spiritual, and physical health along with those we accumulated along the way.

*Illness involves a process* of self-recovery — bursting out of old patterns and developing new ones that serve our newly created self.

*Illness means viewing* our cup of health challenges as half-full, not half-empty — recognizing that you will experience failed hopes and expectations; however, the experience serves to gain a new healthier perspective.

*Illness forces us* to fearlessly examine the things in our life that are not working — then use that information to build and move on, not beat ourselves up for past choices.

*Illness allows us* the opportunity to recognize that true healing only comes when we fully love and respect who we are and, in turn, learn to set our own standards for what we will and will not accept in our lives.

*Illness gives us* the opportunity to test our creative navigation abilities — finding a new path when suddenly the road we're familiar with comes to a dead end.

*Illness builds* compassion and appreciation — you can't have true compassion and appreciation if you haven't experienced the loss of health.

*Illness helps* us recognize that the only thing we can't afford in life is to be around negative people — negativity is a contagious, oftentimes invisible, illness!

— Gloria Gilbère, ND, DA Hom, PhD

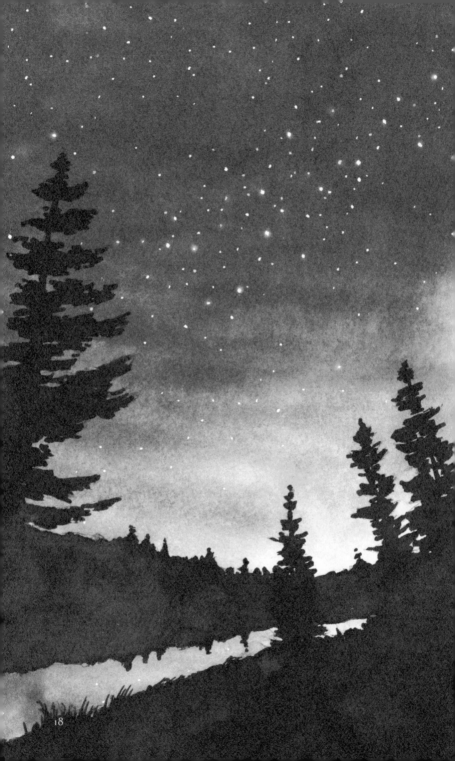

# Some Days Will Be Better Than Others

Some days are better than others.
Some are a little bit worse.
Sometimes everything works out okay.
Sometimes you can't get past the hurts.

When things get a little too stressful and you wonder how you'll make it through, you need to take everything a day at a time, and do what works <u>for you</u>.

Find a place in your heart where you see the way through to the truths about how things can be. Use your inner strength and your quiet resolve and all your positive qualities. Know that you're in the prayers of others. Whisper a few of your own.

You're a strong and special person. The very best is wished for you. Have faith that tomorrow will bring brighter days.

— Marin McKay

# To All Those of Us

To all those of us strapped down by pain
And the world's view of us.

To all those of us
Who have been pushed to the very fringes and beyond,
So that they are nothing but dust,
Shot down in midflight,
To be found too late, too late,
Ragged of skin and broken.

To all those of us
Whose illness isn't painted on the outside of their bodies,
So that it is ignored, argued away, misunderstood.

To all those of us
Whose lives depend to the skin, to the flesh, to the pores,
To the eyes, to the mind, to the senses,
To the very cells,
On the kindness of others (or their non-kindness),
On the giving of others (or their not giving),
On the seeing of others (or their non-seeing),
So that sometimes they barely believe that they are visible.

To all those of us
Who are subject to the mood and moment of the other.

To all those of us
Whose flesh and nerves are painted, raw,
On the outside of their bodies,
And yet to the world, their illness is invisible,
Denied, misunderstood, mistreated.

To all those of us
Whose voices are not heard,
For they have no voice,
Who cannot say your name,
Who cannot say their own name,
Who have no speech,
Who have no words,
And there are no words for this place.

To all those of us
Whose hands used to brandish a sword,
Used to grasp a fountain pen,
A paintbrush,
And who could transform an empty canvas
Into a detailed story of shadow and light,
 delicacy and depth, mood and emotion,
Or who could lift a bow to a cello and make others cry,
Whose fingers could turn the stillness
 of those black and white keys
Into the wild insanity of jazz,
The thumping devotion of gospel,
Or the heavy weight of Beethoven
And whose hands now lie motionless, still,
By their sides, unable to grasp, unable to reach out,
Unable to shape, mould, create,
Unable to signal even,
Who once sang from hill tops,
And who now lie pale because they know no sunshine.

May the world turn around for us,
May the world turn around for us,
May the world turn around for us,

Somehow.

         — Wendy Stern

# Acceptance Doesn't Mean "Giving Up"

Learning to accept the fact that you are ill, chronically ill, is essential to being peaceful and to coping creatively. But acceptance for many who are ill with ICI [Invisible Chronic Illness] is hampered by the fear that acceptance means giving in to illness and, therefore, giving up any attempt to live fully....

But true acceptance never means "giving up"....

Thus, accepting being ill with ICI means knowing yourself, knowing when to rest and when to work, when to play and when to watch, when to exert energy and when to conserve it. Acceptance means admitting the truth of being sick or tired and then deciding what action is most beneficial. It means having the courage to admit at times that you can't do it, whatever the *it* is, and the courage to say no.

— Paul J. Donoghue, PhD and Mary E. Siegel, PhD

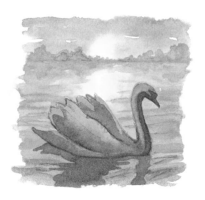

Acceptance means that you
    can find the serenity within
to let go of the past
    with its mistakes and regrets,
move into the future
    with a new perspective,
and appreciate the opportunity
    to take a second chance.

Acceptance means that when
    difficult times come into your life,
you'll find security again and comfort
    to relieve any pain.
You'll find new dreams, fresh hopes,
    and forgiveness of the heart.

Acceptance does not mean
   that you will always be perfect.
It simply means that
   you'll always overcome imperfection.

Acceptance is the road to peace —
   letting go of the worst,
holding on to the best,
   and finding the hope inside
that continues throughout life.

Acceptance is the heart's best defense,
   love's greatest asset,
and the easiest way to keep believing
   in yourself and others.

— Regina Hill

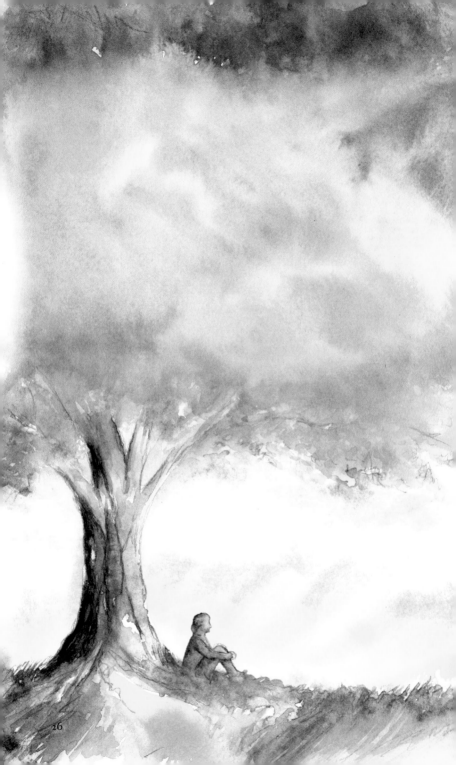

# Only You Know
# What's Right for You

So many choices
So many voices
People tugging a little
People pulling a little
Who to listen to?
Which way to go?
Everyone means well
The sounds are thunderous
The ideas are divergent
The only voice
that must matter
is the one that
resonates in your own heart
The only choice
that must matter
is the one that
you decide is right for you
Only you can decide what
the fabric of your life will be

— Susan Polis Schutz

# Trust Your Instincts

More than anything else, it's essential that you trust your own instincts. You will be relying on your instincts to help guide you toward the practitioners, approaches, and treatments that make the most sense to you. Your decisions may not be made on anything more than a gut feeling, or a sense, after reading or hearing about a particular approach, that "Wow, that just sounds so *right!*" Or you may choose to find a practitioner who inspires your utmost trust, confidence, faith, and hope, and follow his or her direction. Instinct comes into play there as well, because some of the best practitioners are combining their own instincts, applying the "art" of medicine to making decisions about a complex and rarely clear-cut treatment approach.

Trust yourself, trust your instincts, and trust what your body is trying to tell you.

— Mary J. Shomon

Inside of you lie all the answers.
All the worries and confusion you harbor
    as you walk through your life each day
don't have to weigh you down
    and close you off from the true you...
because all the answers lie
    within your soul.

Listen to your heart.
Hear your spirit as it guides you
to the next positive step toward
    your freedom.
Hear your mind's voice leading you
    in the right direction.
You will never lead yourself wrong.

— Paula Michele Adams

# You're Making Progress with Every Step You Take

There are times in life when everything seems to fall apart. Tears and a million pieces of your heart are all that you have to offer, and not enough time has passed to start the healing process.

You long to be rescued from the hurt that is deep inside you, but you know that you can't escape it that easily. Yet somehow, you take a single step forward. It's just a small one — but it is a step.

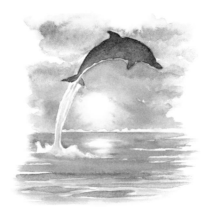

And as the days progress, you will take more —
some without even realizing it — until you've
taken enough to look back and realize that you
have moved forward. Along the way, you will
have picked up some of those broken pieces of
your heart and put them back together again.

Even though it's hard to imagine now, you will be
stronger and braver than before.

— Cody Kohel

# What You Are Doing Takes Real Courage

Courage is the feeling that you can make it,
no matter how challenging the situation.
It is knowing that you can reach out
for help and you are not alone.
Courage is accepting each day,
knowing that you have the inner resources
to deal with the ordinary things
as well as the confusing things,
with the exciting things
as well as the painful things.
Courage is taking the time
to get involved with life, family,
and friends,
and giving your love and energy
in whatever ways you can.

Courage is being who you are,
being aware of your good qualities
and talents,
and not worrying about
what you do not have.
Courage is allowing yourself to live
as fully as you can,
to experience as much of life
as you are able to,
to grow and develop yourself
in whatever directions you need to.
Courage is having hope for the future
and trust in the natural flow of life.
It is being open to change.
Courage is having faith that life
is a beautiful gift.

— Donna Levine-Small

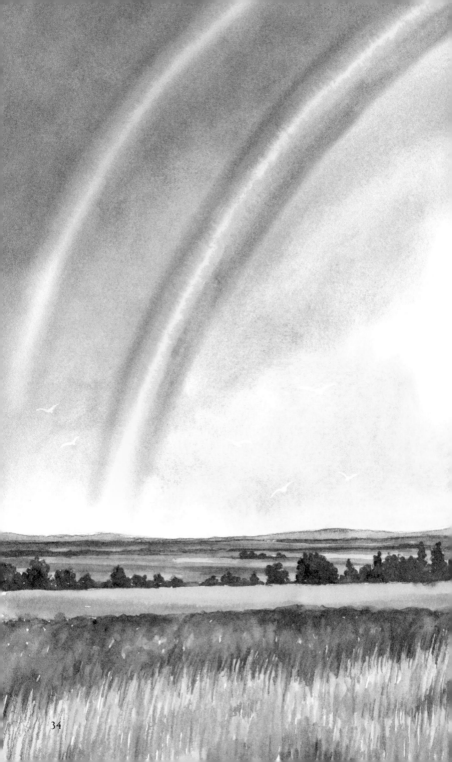

# Believe in the Best Possible Outcome

To attract healthy results, use your attitude of persistence and determination. Every positive thought will signal to your immune system that you are on your own side. Hopeful and faithful statements to yourself will boost your desire and potential to believe in the best outcome you can imagine.

If doubts start to gang up on you, stand up to them. Divert your attention to focus on the most empowering conclusion possible. See yourself with restored energy and pain-free days.

— Donna Fargo

# Take a Deep Breath...

Close your eyes, count to ten,
    and imagine better days.
Imagine your life without
    so many problems.
Picture reaching that point of
    absolute peace.
Erase all your thoughts;
    empty your mind completely.
Take a deep breath and know
nothing is as bad as it seems.

Don't let your current situation trick you
        into believing
that it will be this way forever.
As surely as the sun rises,
        you will have a new day.
You just have to be patient and focus —
not on what you see, but what you
        will soon see.
Believe that better times will arrive.
Believe that you will overcome
what seemed at first to be insurmountable.
Just take a deep breath.

        — Chessica Luckett

# Let It All Go

Let go...
  of guilt; it's okay to make
  the same mistakes again.
Let go...
  of obsessions; they seldom
  turn out the way you planned.
Let go...
  of hate; it's a waste of love.
Let go...
  of blaming others; you are
  responsible for your own destiny.
Let go...
  of fantasies; so reality can
  come true.
Let go...
  of self-pity; someone else may
  need you.
Let go...
  of wanting; cherish what you have.

Let go…
      of fear; it's a waste of faith.
Let go…
      of despair; change comes from
      acceptance and forgiveness.
Let go…
      of the past; the future is
      here — right now.

                    — Kathleen O'Brien

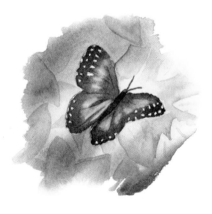

# Hold On to the Good Things in Life

Life continues around us,
even when our troubles seem to stop time.
There is good in life every day.
Take a few minutes to distract yourself
from your concerns —
long enough to draw strength from a tree
or to find pleasure in a bird's song.
Return a smile;
realize that life is a series of levels,
cycles of ups and downs —
some easy, some challenging.

Through it all, we learn;
we grow strong in faith;
we mature in understanding.
The difficult times are often
the best teachers, and there is
good to be found in all situations.
Reach for the good.
Be strong, and don't give up.

— Pamela Owens Renfro

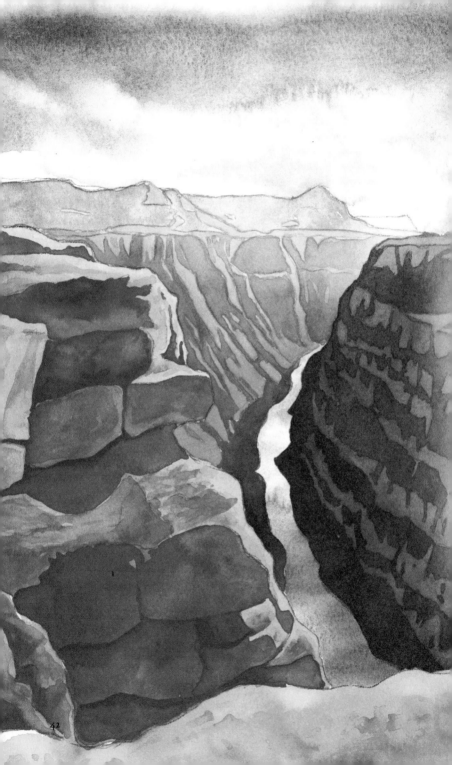

# No One Expects You
# to Have It
# All Figured Out

You don't have to have all the answers or always know the right thing to say. You can climb the highest mountain if you want... or quietly imagine that you might someday. You can take chances or take safety nets, make miracles or make mistakes. You don't have to be composed at all hours to be strong. You don't have to be bold or certain to be brave.

— Ashley Rice

# Just Do Your Best

It's not always easy to know which path to follow, which decision to make, or what to do.

Life is a series of new horizons, new hopes, new days, and changes that come to you. And we all need some help with these things from time to time.

Be positive, for your attitude will affect the outcome of many things. Ask for help when you need it; seek the wisdom the world holds and hold on to it. Make some progress every single day. Begin. Believe. And become.

Give yourself all the credit you're due; don't shortchange your qualities, your abilities, or any of the things that are so unique about you. Remember how precious life can be. Imagine. Invest the time it takes to reach out for your dreams; it will bring you happiness that no money on earth can buy. Don't be afraid to go through life at your own pace.

What's the best thing to do? That's simple:
        Do your best.
And everything else will fall into place.

— Collin McCarty

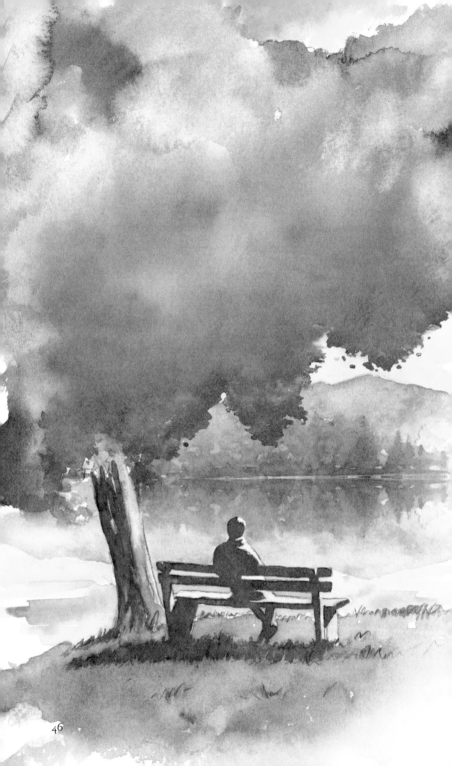

# Make Yourself a Priority

At any given moment on any given day, you are needed. Needed to talk... to drive... to sing... to dance... to laugh... to listen... to help... to walk... to do... something. You say you'll make time for yourself when things slow down, but things will never slow down unless you allow them to.

There will always be that something waving in the background relentlessly trying to get your attention. It's up to you to turn your back... shut your eyes... walk in the opposite direction of that something that just refuses to give you a break. Take the time you deserve to check in with yourself and see what you need for a change.

Be completely and utterly selfish, and do not let guilt creep into your sacred space. No, it's not easy, which is why you have to commit to making a conscious effort to concentrate solely on yourself and your needs. Say no. Turn off your phone. Lock your door to the world. Do whatever it takes to make yourself the ultimate priority.

— Elle Mastro

# Respect Yourself, Respect Your Efforts

This journey isn't easy and it's not for the faint of heart. It takes tremendous courage to allow your suffering, to show genuine compassion for yourself, and to respect yourself for what you have endured. As you've learned by now, not everyone in your pre-illness life will make the journey with you. But at the same time, you've met some very important new people — those who are sharing your journey because they're ill too, or people who like you for who you are and therefore want to share your journey.

No matter how you construct or conceive it, faith is essential to your trip. And the most essential pillar of that faith must be your faith in yourself. This faith will grow as you acquire the ability to see and understand your situation, as you learn how to cope with your particular needs and desires, as you discover the authentic person you are now, and as you learn to tolerate the chronic and the ambiguous. Faith doesn't come with flashes of lightning, huge breakthroughs, or amazing epiphanies. If something like that happens to you, enjoy the experience. But the real growth of faith happens like all growth in nature, slowly, over time. Real faith emerges gradually out of your many small, daily acts of courage when you stand with yourself.

If you feel shaky, remember that you're not alone. Sooner or later, all of us will be on this journey just like you are. You already know people on the road who want to support you, just as you want to support them. Everyone needs to borrow the strength and faith of others at times, just as everyone shares faith and support when they're feeling strong and confident.

— Patricia A. Fennell, MSW, LCSW-R

# Give Friends and Family the Opportunity to Support You

Ask for help.
Whether you need a hand
with running errands or washing dishes...
or you just want some company,
never hesitate to reach out
to family and friends.
Allowing those who love you
to rally around you will lighten your load
and warm their hearts.

— Ali Sawyer

Friends and family are most important. During your most difficult moments and exciting triumphs, they stand beside you. Keep them with you always. They will make life's journey much more rich and rewarding, not to mention fun.

— Donna Gephart

# Help Others Know What Not to Say...

## Fifteen Things Not to Say to Someone with a Chronic Illness or Invisible Illness

1. You don't look sick.
2. You're too young to be sick.
3. Everyone gets tired.
4. You're just having a bad day.
5. It must be nice not having to go to work/school.
6. You need to get more exercise.
7. I wish I had time to take a nap.
8. The power of positive thinking.
9. Just push through it.
10. It will get better, just be patient.
11. Have you tried _____?
12. You should stop _____.
13. It's all in your head. You're just stressed/depressed/anxious.
14. You need to get out more.
15. You take too many medications.

— Susie Helford

# ...and How to Encourage You

## Ten Things You Should Say to Someone with a Chronic Illness

1. I believe you.
2. Can I come over and hang out?
3. Can I bring you food? or, Can I come over and help out around the house?
4. I know how hard you are trying.
5. Any kind of hello or checking in after not seeing them for a while.
6. You are so strong.
7. I know how hard this was for you. Thanks for using your energy to spend time with me.
8. Don't feel bad if you have to cancel plans at the last minute; I understand.
9. Sometimes the best thing you can say is nothing — just a hug or lending an ear.
10. I know this isn't your fault.

BONUS: When all else fails and you aren't sure what to say: I wish I knew what to say, but I care about you, and I'm here for you.

— Susie Helford

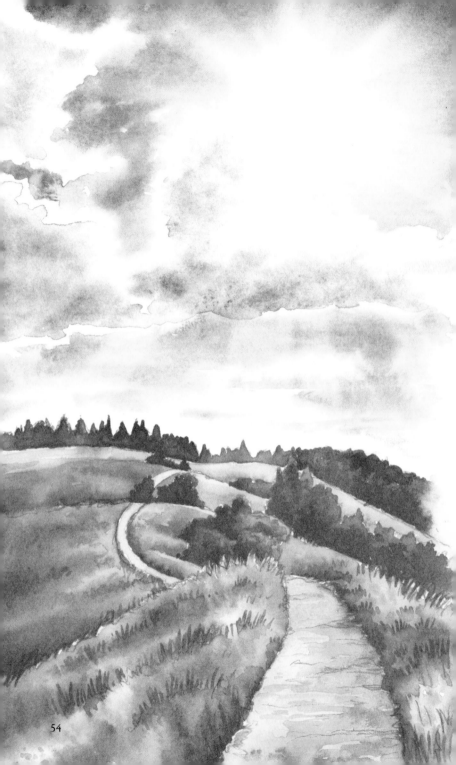

# Talk About
# What You're Feeling

Good or bad, feelings need expression;
they must be recognized and given
freedom to reveal themselves.
It isn't wise to hide behind a smile
when your heart is breaking;
that is not being true to how
you feel inside.

Put away the myth that says
you must be strong enough
to face the whole world with a smile
and a brave attitude all the time.
You have your feelings that say otherwise,
so admit that they are there.
Use their healing power
to put the past behind you,
and realize those expressive
stirrings in your heart
are very much a part of you.
Use them to find peace within
and to be true to yourself.

— Barbara J. Hall

# It's Okay...

It's okay to be afraid
of the things you don't understand.
It's okay to feel anxious
when things aren't working your way.
It's okay to feel lonely...
even when you're with other people.
It's okay to feel unfulfilled
because you know something is missing
(even if you're not sure what it is).
It's okay to think and worry and cry.

It's okay to do
whatever you have to do,
but just remember, too,
that eventually you're going to adjust
to the changes life brings your way,
and you'll get to the point where
the life you live is full and
satisfying and good to you…
and it will be that way
because you made it that way.

— Laine Parsons

# Sometimes You Just Need to Walk Away

Sometimes
it is all just too much
too much to fathom
too much to analyze
too much to accept
too much to do

Sometimes
it is better to just let go
of all the problems
of all the tasks
of all the burdens
that weigh you down

Sometimes
the greatest gift you can
    give yourself
is to walk away
to walk out from under
to walk into sunshine
    and warm your soul

Sometimes
you will return
and your burdens will seem
somehow easier to handle
    than before

Rest in the assuredness
that you are enough after all

— Minx Boren, MCC

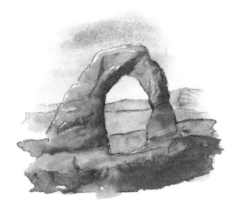

# The War Inside
# My Body

There is a war inside my body.
My brain explodes with bombshells of pain,
the fog of the frontline never clears.
My muscles fire their artilleries
as the dictator feeds on them.
My blood and my heart beat on, beat on,
passing resources along the supply chain,
hoping they are not stolen
by the marauding enemy.
My immune system is under siege,
surrounded and weakening day by day.

But the dictator doesn't understand that
if I weaken, so does he,
the more he destroys, destroys, destroys.
The dictator only sees the present.
He only wants to survive NOW —
to see *his* children flourish
in a ripe and supple landscape
that shrivels and decays the longer he resides here.
Me — my own muscles, my brain, my blood —
overrun and oppressed
subdued and subjected.

This war is painfully intense,
and it feels as if victory will surely be his.
But I will fight for freedom
so that verdant things, healthy things, fertile things
grow in my heart, my flesh, my mind once more.
Someday,
I will run along the pathways of the earth,
and my imagination will fly amongst starlit skies,
and the war inside my body
will be no more.

— Teryn O'Brien

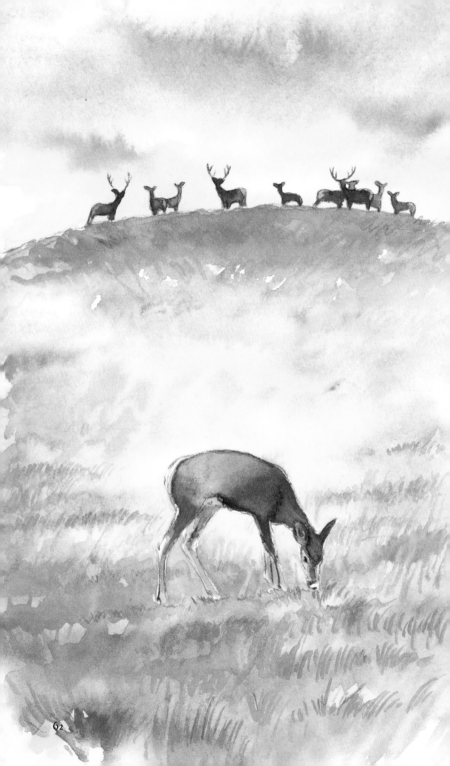

# When You Need Some Help to Get Through...

When nothing is going right.
When you're wondering,
    "What did I do to deserve this?"
When the day is a disaster
and a little serenity
    is just what you're after.
When you need a whole lot less
    to concern you
and a whole lot more to smile about.
When a few peaceful hours
    would seem like a vacation to you
and you're wondering if there's anything
    you've got to look forward to...
Sometimes you just have to remember:
    You're going to make it
        through this day.
    Even if it's one step at a time.
Sometimes you just have to be
    patient and brave and strong.
If you don't know how,
    just make it up as you go along.

— Collin McCarty

# What I've Learned

Learning to accept and live with
  limitations
by a person who thought they didn't
  have any
is difficult yet vital
I learned that
everyone has something that stops them
and you just have to circumvent these
right now
because one day
any day
everything stops
Life stops
Understanding the fragility of my breath
I decided to inhale deeply in gratitude
I learned
how to have different ways of having joy

I can't walk on the beach
but I can dig in the sand
I can't run around the bases
but I can watch the games
I can't move very fast
but I can still think fast
I can't plant flowers
but I can smell them
So many things I can't do
yet so many things I can do
And best of all
I can love
with no limitations
with all the passion I've ever had
And that's the
most gratifying and meaningful music
of all humanity

— Susan Polis Schutz

# Keep Faith
# in Your Heart

With faith, you can move a mountain,
reach a star,
and make it through the longest night.

With faith, you can trust
that everything has a reason
and every life a purpose —
you can feel content
with what you have
and stay secure within yourself.

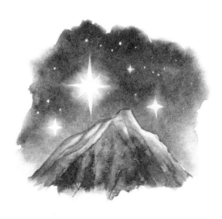

With faith, you can look back
on your most trying time
and see it for the blessing it was —
an experience that led you
where you were meant to go
and helped shape the person
you were created to be.

With faith, you can look
for the bright side
of any situation…
and always find it.

— Paula Finn

# Find Hope Within

Hope is such a marvelous thing.
It bends, it twists, it sometimes hides,
but rarely does it break.

Hope sustains us when nothing else can.
It gives us reason to continue
and the courage to move ahead
when we tell ourselves
we'd rather give in.

Hope puts smiles on our faces
when our hearts cannot manage.
Hope puts our feet on the path
when our eyes cannot see it.
Hope moves us to act when our souls
are confused by the direction.

Hope is a wonderful thing —
something to be cherished and nurtured
and that will refresh us in return.
It can be found in each of us,
and it can bring light into
the darkest of places.

— Brenda Hager

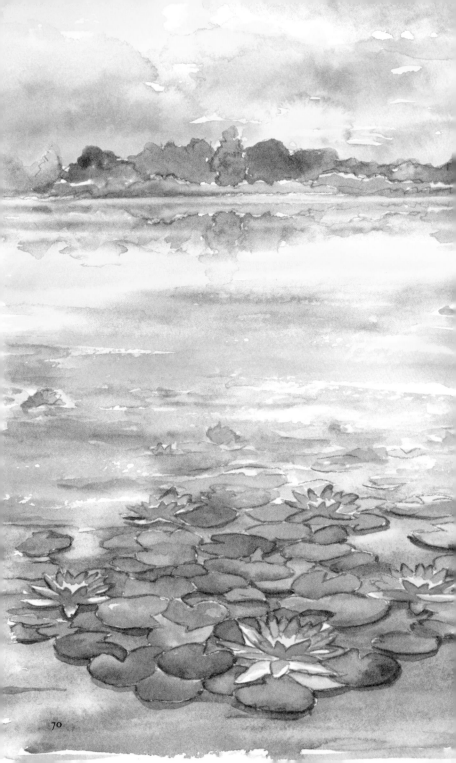

# Focus on
# the Present

We cannot change the past;
we just need to keep
the good memories
and acquire wisdom
from the mistakes we've made.
We cannot predict the future;
we just need to hope and pray
for the best and what is right
and believe that's how it will be.
We can live a day at a time,
enjoying the present
and always seeking to become
a more loving and better person.

— Karen Berry

# Remember What Is Most Important...

It's not having everything go right;
it's facing whatever goes wrong.
It's not being without fear;
it's having the determination
     to go on in spite of it.

What is most important is not
     where you stand,
but the direction you're going in.
It's more than never having bad moments;
it's knowing you are always
     bigger than the moment.
It's believing you have already
     been given everything
you need to handle life.

It's not being able to rid
    the world of all its injustices;
it's being able to rise above them.
It's the belief in your heart
    that there will always be
more good than bad in the world.

Remember to live just this one day
and not add tomorrow's troubles
    to today's load.
Remember that every day ends
and brings a new tomorrow
full of exciting new things.
Love what you do,
    do the best you can,
and always remember
    how much you are loved.

— Vickie M. Worsham

# Make Every Day Special

Make every day a day to celebrate life and be thankful. Take time to pull yourself away from all the noise and just look around you.

Take inventory. Appreciate those who have enhanced the quality of your life, and remember that they have been a gift to you. Also remember that you're a gift to them too.

Be grateful for the choices you've made, both good and bad. Accept your mistakes; you can't change them anyway. Appreciate yourself and your own uniqueness.

Go outside and look at the sky. Soak in the atmosphere. Enjoy the colors of the landscape. Feel the textures of every place you are that you're thankful for. Smile at the world.

Don't allow any negative feelings to creep into your consciousness. Feel the power of your own acceptance. Put a positive spin on every thought you have.

Make every day special. Own it. Enjoy it. Bask in the glory of life. Appreciate the gift of your own life.

— Donna Fargo

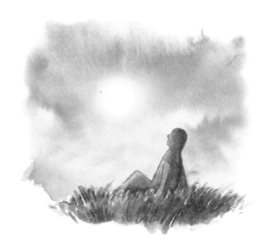

# Eleven "Don'ts" for Living with Chronic Illness

Don't let go of hope.
Hope gives you the strength
to keep going
when you feel like giving up.
Don't ever quit believing in yourself.
As long as you believe you can,
you will have a reason for trying.
Don't let anyone hold your happiness
in their hands;
hold it in yours
so it will always be within your reach.
Don't measure success or failure
by material wealth,
but by how you feel;
our feelings determine
the richness of our lives.
Don't let bad moments overcome you;
be patient, and they will pass.

Don't hesitate to reach out for help;
we all need it from time to time.
Don't run away from love but toward love,
because it is our deepest joy.
Don't wait for what you want
to come to you.
Go after it with all that you are,
knowing that life will meet you halfway.
Don't feel like you've lost
when plans and dreams fall short
    of your hopes.
Anytime you learn something new
about yourself or about life,
you have progressed.
Don't do anything that takes away
from your self-respect.
Feeling good about yourself
is essential to feeling good about life.
Don't ever forget how to laugh
or be too proud to cry.
It is by doing both
that we live life to its fullest.

— Nancye Sims

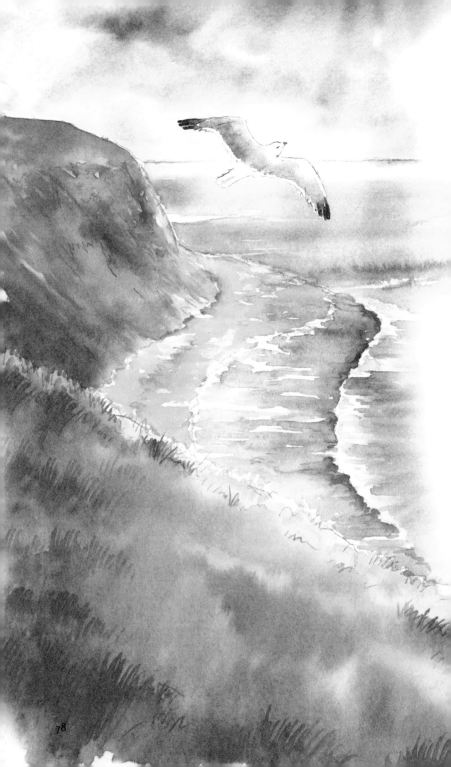

# You Are a Survivor

There will be times when you're going to need so much courage. There will be times when you'll feel like crying yourself to sleep... when your confidence is shaken... when you're scared, angry, and confused... when you can't believe this is happening to you.

But for every one of those situations, there will also be times when you look deep inside and realize... you're going to be okay.

There will be times when you find out that you're such a fighter... when you discover how strong you really can be and that you're truly a survivor.

— Terry Bairnson

Nobody ever said that it would be easy or that the skies would always be sunny. When gray days and worrisome times come along, you need to stay strong.

When life has got you down, remember: it's all right to feel vulnerable. You feel things deeply, and that is a wonderful quality to have. Rest assured that, in the long run, the good days will outnumber the bad.

What is sometimes perceived as weakness is actually strength. The more you're bothered by something that's wrong, the more you're empowered to make things right. Each day is like a room you spend time in before you move on to the next. And in each room — filled with possibilities — there is a door that leads to more serenity in life.

Leave behind any little worries. Tomorrow they won't matter, and next month you may not even remember what they were. Take the others one at a time, and you'll be amazed at how your difficulties manage to become easier.

Find your smile. Warm yourself with your quiet determination and your knowledge of brighter days ahead. Do the things that need to be done. Say the words that need to be said.

Happiness is waiting for you. Believe in your ability. Cross your bridges. Listen to your heart. Your faith in tomorrow will always help you do what is right… and it will help you be strong.

— Collin McCarty

# This Can Be a
# Time of Growth

As difficult as this time in your life may be,
you will become stronger if you
face each day with patience and hope;
if you accept your weaknesses
but concentrate on your strengths;
if you love and care for yourself
even when you are angry and confused;
if you can look at doubt and fear
but keep your mind on the fact that
the struggle is helping you to grow
   in faith and confidence.

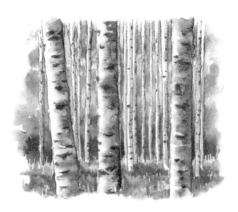

If you gently pick yourself up when you fall
and continue walking;
if you keep thinking about
all the things you can do well,
all the things that bring you joy,
and all the people you love who also love you;
if you hold on to your goals
even though the way to reach them
    may be unclear, then…

You can see the troubling times
almost as friends who have come
to help you grow further
than you thought you could;
friends who are showing you the way
to a more courageous heart;
friends who help you to see that
you are more powerful than
you ever thought you were;
friends who help you to see that
the hard times are making you more open
to accepting life as it comes
and realizing that you have
the inner strength and loving nature
to deal successfully with any difficult moment.

— Donna Levine-Small

# You Have the Power

Have patience
with yourself and the situation.
Live in the moment, one day at a time,
not fretting about the past
    or worrying about the future.
You have strength enough for the present,
and that is all you need for now.
Allow yourself the luxury of peace,
and don't take on more than you have to.
Learn to let go.
Refuse negative thoughts;
replace them with positive ones.
Look for the good things in your life,
and make a point to appreciate them.

Believe in yourself and know
     that you have the power.
You are ultimately the one
     in charge of your life
and the only person in the world
     who can change it.
No matter how much others
     are pulling for you
or how much anyone else cares,
<u>you</u> must do what needs to be done
to make your present and future
everything you want and
     need it to be.
                    — Barbara Cage

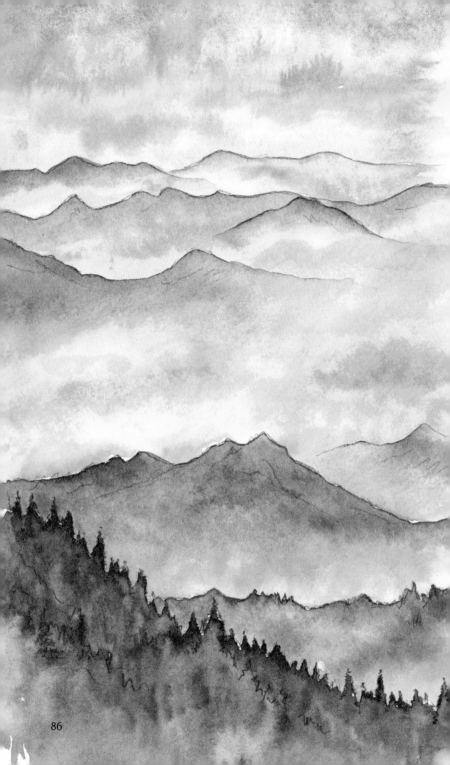

# Take It One Day
# at a Time

Sometimes in life we don't know where to begin, but if we take a step back, we can gain a different perspective that will remind us to take it one day at a time.

If you feel like you are standing still when all you want to do is hit the ground running, just remember that things take time and patience is key.

As long as you are placing one foot in front of the other and keeping your focus, you will find the answers you so desperately seek. You may even find that some truly great opportunities come to you in your patience.

Take it one day at a time, and as long as you do, you will make progress.

— Lamisha Serf-Walls

# Know That You'll Make It Through

How do you make it through? You face your fears. You keep your promises. You deal directly with your challenges. You get the best possible help and care. You turn to caring, positive people you know will be there for you.

You believe. You take steps to change what needs changing. You talk it over. You laugh. You go ahead and cry. You pray. You stay involved. You live the best life you can today. And when tomorrow comes, you do it all over again.

You hang in there. You hold on tight to your hope. You never let go. You know, deep down inside, what a special person you are. And no matter what comes along, you never forget it. You stay strong. You keep the faith. And you make room for the brighter day that, someday soon, is going to shine so much serenity back into your life.

— Anna Tafoya

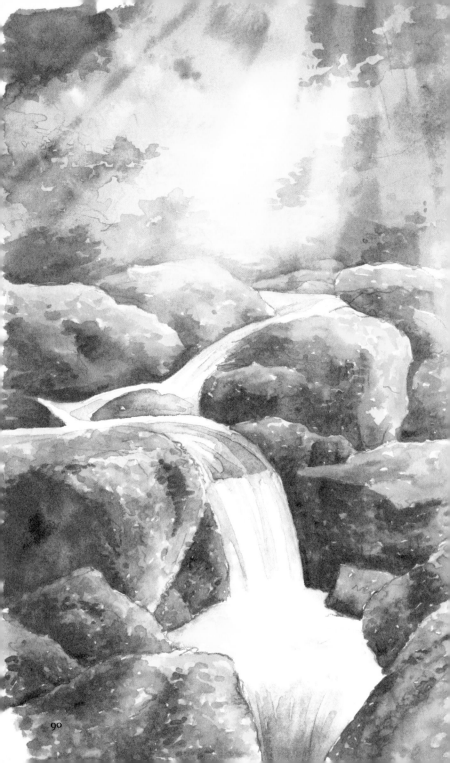

# May Faith, Courage, and Hope Help You Through Even the Hardest Days

When life seems like a mountain
that's too hard to climb...
    may you find the strength
        to take just one more step.
When your journey seems just
too hard to bear...
    may you find the courage
        to face one more day.
When you feel lost and you don't know
    which way to turn...
        may your faith and trust
        lead the way.
And when it's hard to believe
    that things will ever get better...
    may you look inside your heart —
    and find hope.

— Jason Blume

# ACKNOWLEDGMENTS

We gratefully acknowledge the permission granted by the following authors, publishers, and authors' representatives to reprint poems or excerpts in this publication:

PrimaDonna Entertainment Corp. for "Make every day a day to celebrate life...," "As you dodge the curve balls...," and "To attract healthy results..." by Donna Fargo. Copyright © 1998, 2005, 2016 by PrimaDonna Entertainment Corp. All rights reserved. Nancye Sims for "When the challenges seem so much greater...." Copyright © 2016 by Nancye Sims. All rights reserved. Gloria Gilbère, ND, DA Hom, PhD for "Illness, especially when it's invisible..." from INVISIBLE ILLNESSES. Copyright © 2002, 2005 by Gloria Gilbère, ND, DA Hom, PhD. All rights reserved. Malcom Stern for "To All Those of Us" by Wendy Stern. Copyright © 2014 by Wendy Stern. All rights reserved. W. W. Norton & Company, Inc., for "Learning to accept the fact..." from SICK AND TIRED OF FEELING SICK AND TIRED: LIVING WITH INVISIBLE CHRONIC ILLNESS by Paul J. Donoghue, PhD and Mary E. Siegel, PhD. Copyright © 1992 by Paul J. Donoghue and Mary E. Siegel. All rights reserved. HarperCollins Publishers for "Trust Your Instincts" from LIVING WELL WITH CHRONIC FATIGUE SYNDROME AND FYBROMYALGIA by Mary J. Shomon. Copyright © 2004 by Mary J. Shomon. All rights reserved. Paula Michele Adams for "Inside of you lie all the answers." Copyright © 2016 by Paula Michele Adams. All rights reserved. Cody Kohel for "There are times in life when...." Copyright © 2016 by Cody Kohel. All rights reserved. Donna Levine-Small for "Courage is the feeling that you can make it...." Copyright © 2016 by Donna Levine-Small. All rights reserved. Chessica Luckett for "Close your eyes, count to ten...." Copyright © 2016 by Chessica Luckett. All rights reserved. New Harbinger Publications, Inc., for "Respect Yourself, Respect Your Efforts" from THE CHRONIC ILLNESS WORKBOOK by Patricia A. Fennell, MSW, LCSW-R. Copyright © 2001 by Patricia A. Fennell. All rights reserved. Susie Helford for "Fifteen Things Not to Say..." and "Ten Things You Should Say..." from Pins and Procrastination (blog), April 15, 2014 and May 13, 2014, http://www.pinsandprocrastination.com. Copyright © 2014 by Susie Helford. All rights reserved. Barbara J. Hall for "Good or bad, feelings need expression...." Copyright © 2016 by Barbara J. Hall. All rights reserved. Minx Boren for "Sometimes it is all just too much..." from HEALING IS A JOURNEY. Copyright © 2014 by Minx Boren. All rights reserved. Teryn O'Brien, www.terynobrien.com, for "The War Inside My Body." Copyright © 2015 by Teryn O'Brien. All rights reserved. Paula Finn for "With faith, you can move a mountain...." Copyright © 2016 by Paula Finn. All rights reserved. Brenda Hager for "Hope is such a marvelous thing." Copyright © 2016 by Brenda Hager. All rights reserved. Lamisha Serf-Walls for "Sometimes in life we don't know...." Copyright © 2016 by Lamisha Serf-Walls. All rights reserved. Jason Blume for "When life seems like a mountain...." Copyright © 2008 by Jason Blume. All rights reserved.

A careful effort has been made to trace the ownership of selections used in this anthology in order to obtain permission to reprint copyrighted material and give proper credit to the copyright owners. If any error or omission has occurred, it is completely inadvertent, and we would like to make corrections in future editions provided that written notification is made to the publisher:

BLUE MOUNTAIN ARTS, INC., P.O. Box 4549, Boulder, Colorado 80306.